T0197472

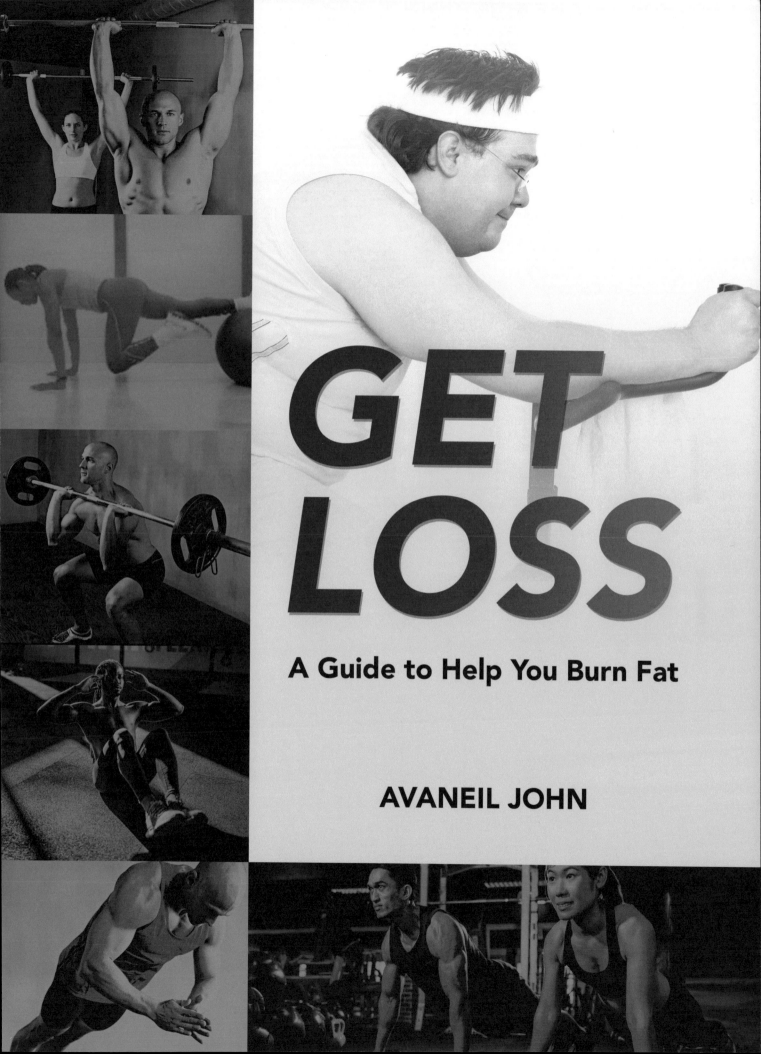

GET LOSS

A Guide to Help You Burn Fat

AVANEIL JOHN

GET LOSS

A Guide to Help You Burn Fat

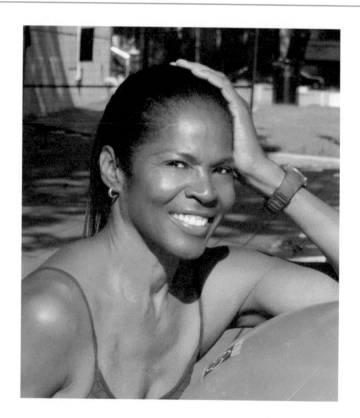

AVANEIL JOHN

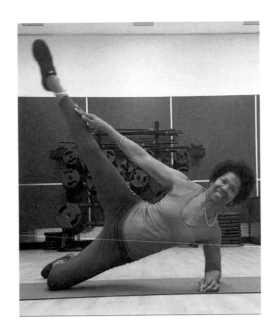

AuthorHouse™
1663 Liberty Drive
Bloomington, IN 47403
www.authorhouse.com
Phone: 1 (833) 262-8899

Because of the dynamic nature of the Internet, any web addresses or links contained in this book may have changed
since publication and may no longer be valid. The views expressed in this work are solely those of the author and do not
necessarily reflect the views of the publisher, and the publisher hereby disclaims any responsibility for them.

Any people depicted in stock imagery provided by Getty Images are models,
and such images are being used for illustrative purposes only.
Certain stock imagery © Getty Images.

This book is printed on acid-free paper.

ISBN: 978-1-7283-7155-9 (sc)
ISBN: 978-1-7283-7156-6 (e)

Print information available on the last page.

Published by AuthorHouse 08/19/2021

authorHOUSE®

DISCLAIMER

This book is not intended as a substitute for the medical advice of physicians or health practitioners. The content is to inform and educate the reader. Before commencing any weight reduction or nutritional program, the reader should consult a physician in matters relating to his or her health and particularly any symptoms that may require diagnosis or medical attention.

You are cautioned to rely on your own judgment about your individual health circumstances and act accordingly at your own risk when applying the content of this book. This book makes no claims or guarantees that you will lose body fat under your own volition. Not everyone will lose fat at the same rate because every individual is biochemically different.

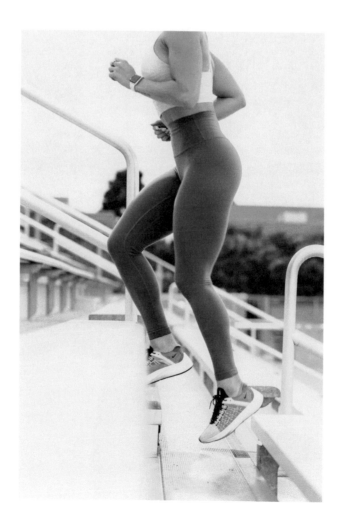

ACKNOWLEDGEMENT

It is great to have friends, but it is even greater when they take an interest in what you do and vice versa. Therefore, I cannot express enough my gratitude to Atherton Leatham, nutritionist; Dirk McLean, author; and Novia John, university professor, for taking time from their busy schedule to read and provide feedback for this book.

Also, thanks to Unsplash for some great photographs.

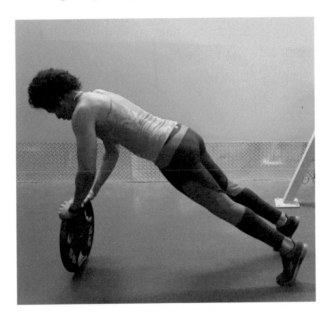

CONTENTS

*"You cannot buy good health to live a healthier lifestyle.
But you can create a healthier lifestyle to live in good health."*
Avaneil John

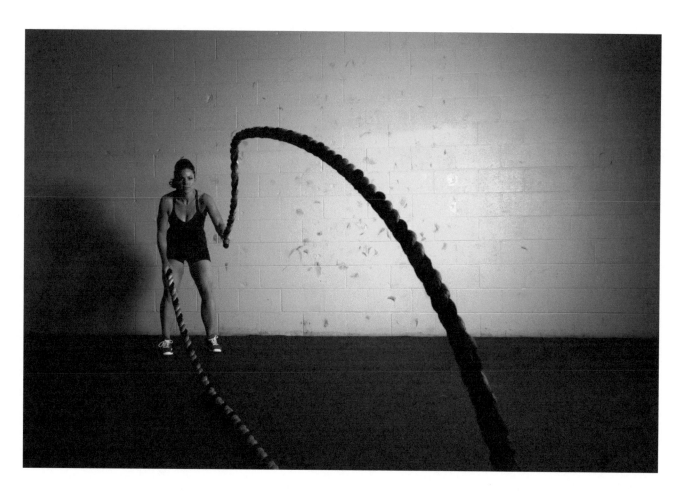

INTRODUCTION

This book provides a synopsis of information that is highly valuable for a person in approaching the shedding of unwanted accumulated pounds. Fat loss should be achieved wisely—especially as a beginner. Many people are seen attempting fat loss without a proper approach, thereby, engaging in unhealthy ways for achieving their goal.

Before we begin our fat loss program, you must understand what is involved. Some individuals are keen to start losing body fat, jumping right into a quick-fix diet or exercise regimen without preparing for the process. Impatient, they bypass the acquiring or gaining of the knowledge for effective fat loss. Their effort then backfires, and they end up in no better shape than what they began with.

Fat loss is a process of healthy and sustainable practices. It is not just about calorie reduction and physical activity, but also involves shifting your mindset to make a healthier lifestyle change.

Your journey may be difficult, but the results can be rewarding. So believe in your vision. Your mind will be flexible with positive thinking.

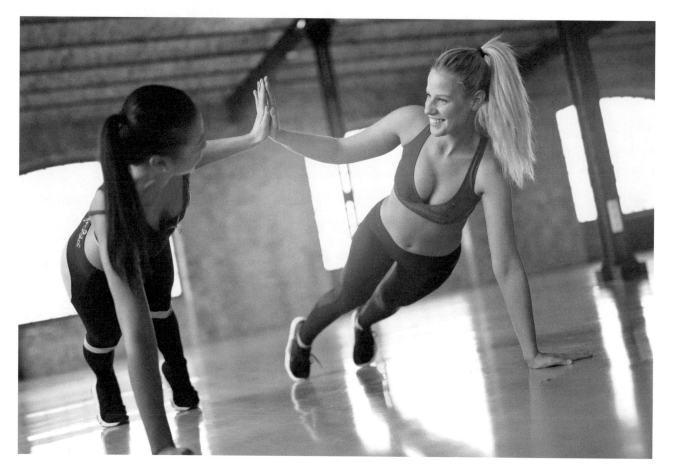

Get in the mindset to lose body fat:

"A positive mindset will drive
Your thoughts to what you will achieve.
It makes you who you become."
Avaneil John

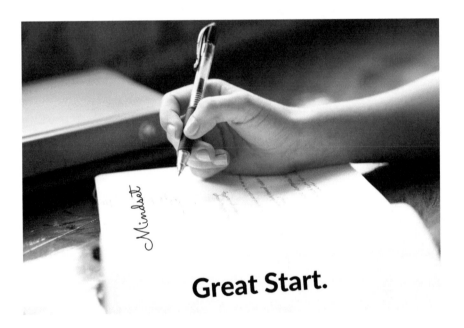

Great Start.

I n this section, we ignite the awareness of the frame-of-mind requirements for understanding the approach to fat loss and how this mindset is achieved.

Before beginning a program, remember that size and beauty are two separate things. Likewise, size and health are also two different things. The first thing you must do is ask yourself, *"What is it that makes me want to change my appearance?"* Do you want a change in body size? Do you not value the beauty that lies within yourself because of the size? Is it to please someone in your life? Are you trying to live up to the societal concepts of beauty? Is it because a doctor recommended it? Is it to overcome physical limitations? Is it to be prepared in making dietary and nutritional changes for a healthier lifestyle? Do you have the mental stamina to apply yourself to a program? Then ask yourself whether you can devote yourself to a sustained program of change. As you ask yourself these questions, answer yourself truthfully to have a better perception of what you truly and honestly want. Because this path should lead to an appreciation of your health journey, it needs to be built on honesty with yourself. Now, the next thing you want to do is consult your doctor regarding this attempt. Be honest. The doctor may have great advice for you, guiding you in the right direction.

There is much more to fat loss than just diet and exercise. There is the mental mindset that involves discipline, determination, commitment, willpower, and patience, all of which are traits that would help you get your desired results. Also, you must know the physical demands that are required—the advantages and disadvantages, the appreciation and the benefits that come with your efforts. Understanding the fundamental principles will set the stage for a successful lifestyle change and fat-loss journey.

Although fat loss might be the result, it should not be a goal because in your eagerness to lose fat quickly, you may opt for "shortcuts." Your goal should be gradual, small and sustainable-healthy lifestyle changes that are in your control. Losing body fat does not happen overnight. It requires staying powerful and may require a range of training methods to achieve the best outcome. An individual attempting to get in shape must be prepared and focused on changing old unhealthy habits and appreciating new healthy ones.

Often, your eagerness may assign a specific time frame to achieve fat loss. It may not happen as you wish—unrealistic expectations may set you up for failure. Everyone does not experience the burning of fat at the same rate. Someone may experience results sooner than others—just like those who give up trying, while others stay on the course. Regardless of the time it takes, just appreciate the benefits it brings along the way, and be grateful for the little steps you take.

Also, it is important to note that your weight may fluctuate. It happens because of the number of calories you consume, your workout regime, and even the amount of sleep you get. For example, eating a salad or even drinking a glass of water will add weight to your body. This is just normal. This understanding will maintain your confidence throughout your efforts.

How to achieve the mindset and be motivated for fat loss:

Thinking of fat loss and taking action towards it are two different things. Both concepts require mindful motivation. You will accomplish this by assessing your motivation and readiness for the change:

- Determine the reason for weight loss. *This will give you a drive/motive.*

- Are you ready or just pre-contemplating fat loss? If you are not prepared, commit to a starting date in your journal: *"I will begin a fat-loss journey on May 1st of this year." This will keep anticipation high.*

- Be enthusiastic. Your enthusiasm will help you commit to a lifestyle change. *It will help prepare you to take action.*

- If you listen to someone else's fat-loss failure, do not let it decrease your positive thoughts; *learn from it. You will know what to avoid. It will help enhance your motivation and mindset.*

- Focus on solutions for achieving your goal—not excuses. *It will help you to be responsible and break through barriers.*

- Surround yourself with positive people; *their environment provides positive energy and encouragement.*

- If you need help to develop your mindset, ask for help. *Personal trainers, psychologists, or life/wellness coaches can help you hone the right state of mind to achieve your goal.*

Now that you have developed the mindset, and your commitment and determination are high—take action. Being mentally ready with a properly planned outline for your journey, you are bound to achieve great results!

*"Work out to enhance who you were meant to be,
not who others think you should be."*
Avaneil John

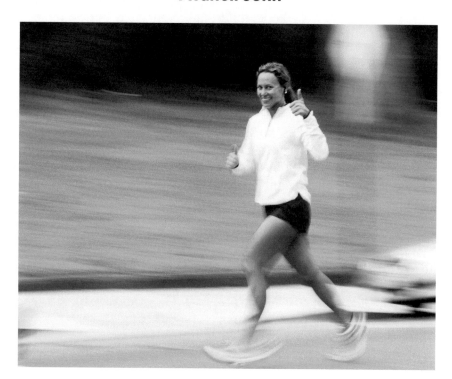

In this section, you will know the difference of weight-reduction variables, setting goals for results, and how to prepare for a direction of nutrition for fat loss:

How to distinguish weight loss vs. fat loss:

Weight Loss is a reduction of total body mass. In other words, the entire components of the body, which includes essential body fat, muscle, bone, fluids, and organ size. For example, when you step on a scale and weigh 10 pounds less, that is the total body-weight loss of all components, including the essential fat—not the non-essential stored fat which we do not need.

This method of weight loss is quick and can fluctuate daily. For instance, if you do not eat or drink all day, you would experience some weight loss—so anyone can lose weight. This progress gives a false sense of losing fat. Weight loss can make you look soft, stretchy, and flabby with a sagging belly.

Fat Loss is a decrease of stored body fat, which is specific to the body fat storage components—a reduction of *only* body fat. You reduce overall body mass by burning the size of stored calories, which takes a longer time to burn while preserving muscle. This is a healthier and sustainable approach.

Knowing the difference between the two components will help you with the aspect of progress.

How to implement long-term and short-term goals of fat loss:

Goals give you focus and allow you to evaluate progress. They can vary from three months to one year or more. When setting goals, there are five S.M.A.R.T. principles to consider:

- **S**pecific: I will lose 10 pounds by doing cardio and consuming healthy meals 6 days a week.

- **M**easurable: I will run/swim on Mondays and Wednesdays from 4:00 to 4:30 p.m. weekly.

- **A**chievable: I will lose 1 to 2 pounds each week.

- **R**elevant: I will lose 10 pounds to decrease potential heart risks.

- **T**imeline: I will lose 10 pounds by March 5th of this year.

Regardless of the long-term or short-term goals, they would determine the period for their achievements. Long-term goals provide purpose, and a path to follow until you achieve your goal. Short-term goals are like stepping stones/baby steps to guide you through your journey to attain results.

For example, if you want to lose 100 pounds in 12 months, this would be your bigger goal. Now that you have this goal in mind, you can set up short-term goals on how to achieve that goal. Short-term goals help you to break down the larger long-term goal. Short-term goals can ensure that you stay motivated.

For instance, a good short-term goal would be to lose 1 pound of fat weekly. Also, determine how you will achieve it. In other words, I will run or walk three miles, three times a week, or weight train twice weekly and consume healthy and well-balanced meals daily. Each weekly short-term achievement will lead you closer to your long-term goal.

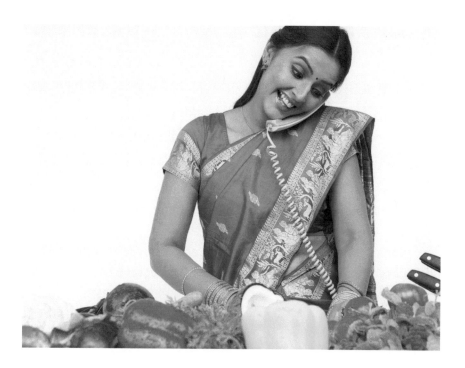

Nutrition Guidelines

Fat loss can be a struggle that many people face, especially when there is constant promotion of food everywhere we turn. Your ability to resist certain foods will be the test along your journey, whether it is at a dinner table or by the enticing advertisements we come across daily.

Weight loss advertising programs:

Advertisements are intended to lure you into their web. Their enticing slogans of diet plans and pills with empty promises to lose weight faster than a speeding bullet is not a healthy approach. According to research, there are over 7,000 pills, powders, and plans available on the market. And guess which one works!? The way to control advertisement enticement is to picture the physique you desire immediately and remember why you are doing it—always keep your eyes on the fat-loss prize.

Before you purchase any weight-loss scheme, ensure that it is right for you. Again, have a quick consultation with your doctor or health practitioner to avoid ingesting any products that may not be right for you.

Ways to cleanse the body:

Your body is an amazing tool that naturally removes impurities on its own. However, its ability to efficiently process toxins is limited if it is overloaded with unhealthy foods and the environmental pollution we deal with. Getting rid of toxins is a good start—a clean slate to introduce your body to healthy habits.

It is best to consider using natural products for cleansing. The best colon cleansers are foods high in dietary fibre. It contributes to cleansing by providing bulk for regular bowel movements. But fibre alone cannot clean the colon. Additionally, I use other natural ingredients. There are two types of fibers: soluble and insoluble, and they both contribute to cleansing, fat loss and maintaining weight without adding many calories to your meal plan. Here is an example of both fibers: an apple, the skin is insoluble and the inside is soluble.

Experts recommend eating some fibre at every meal to spread your intake throughout the day.

For example, when preparing breakfast, I add 100 grams of vanilla yogurt to ½ cup raw (or cooked) 100% whole grain oats; ¼ slice of diced apple; ½ of a small banana chopped; ¼ of a small avocado; (optional: 1 coarsely chopped strawberry and ¼ cup blueberries) and sprinkle 1 teaspoon of hemp seeds on top. This makes for a fibrous and flavorful meal.

Other cleansers are natural herbs. Sometimes, I boil 1 teaspoon Senna Leaves or Senna Roots in 2 cups of water to clean the colon. Caution: if you use these herbs regularly, your system may depend on it for bowel movements. To cleanse the kidneys, I boil ½ cup fresh parsley leaves in 2 cups water; or I prepare 1 teaspoon ginger and/or dandelion root in the same way. For the liver, I boil 1 teaspoon of milk thistle and/or peppermint in 2 cups of water, and simmer herbs for 5-10 minutes. They are all used as tea. If the taste is too pungent, I add ½ teaspoon of honey or maple syrup. Before you use *any* of the cleansing systems, I recommend that you consult with your local herbalist, medical physician, or health practitioner.

Drinking eight glasses of water can help to cleanse your system. You can add half of a fresh lemon juice in the water to give it some flavor and punch. However, based on your size and physical activity, you may consume more water.

Another drink I have used is V-8 juice, which has about 6 grams of fibre. You can add a teaspoon of oats for added fibre and mix it for about 5 seconds in a blender.

Alternatively, there is psyllium husk, which is also used for the cleansing of the system. Psyllium husks thicken quickly. It is best to shake it in a container (stirring thickens it faster), then drink it immediately. If you are not sure what cleansing method would work for you, consult with your medical doctor or health practitioner.

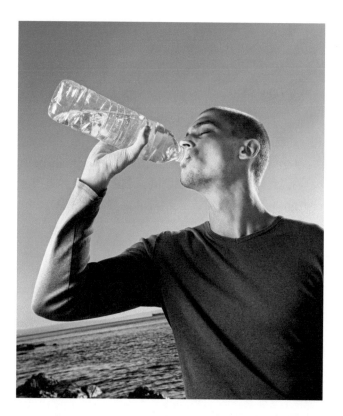

How the digestive system and burning calories could help body fat loss:

**"Results lie in the effort, not in the attainment of your goal.
The test is your persistence for success."**
Avaneil John

When preparing for fat loss, note that although calories are the prime factor for losing fat, it is not as simple as "calories in, calories out." There can be many factors such as the inner workings of the body, namely the digestive system. It plays a significant role when starting a fat-loss program because it is the core for burning fat. Digestion regulates the flow of food. For instance, if you chew food too quickly, large pieces of undigested food will be held in the stomach longer—the food just sits there. This can turn into fat and may induce bloating and constipation, which adds weight to the body.

Further, the digestion and/or metabolism—even the immune system may not function adequately. In other words, the body may not get the benefits of sufficient nutrients—even though you are eating healthy to promote fat loss. Other drawbacks may involve hormone imbalances, metabolism inefficiency, lack of fibre, underlying medical conditions such as hypothyroidism or certain medications.

You may not connect the immune system with fat loss because we believe it helps prevent colds or viruses, and avert other potential illnesses, which is true. But the immune system plays an important role in controlling body weight. *"Have you tried to lose body fat and failed, despite your best efforts to eat healthy and exercise regularly, but the weight refuses to leave?"* The reasons might be the effect of a weak immune system. To burn carbs and promote fat loss, the immune system must function properly.

So, how to improve the digestive and immune system?

Your digestive system will help you lose fat if it is working properly. Digestion is easy to regulate, you have to be patient. Here are a few ways: drink more water, it keeps the flow of food moving through the digestive system; eat more fibre, it helps the digestive tract move stool efficiently; eat slowly, it breaks down food in smaller particles for easier digestion and absorption; workout, it increases your metabolic rate which improves digestion.

You can boost the immune system by consuming green leafy vegetables such as kale, broccoli, cabbage; multi-vitamin and mineral supplements; herbs are also critical for a healthy immune system. For example, I have consulted with my herbalist who suggested these three herbs to improve my immune system: astragalus, echinacea and reishi mushrooms. I boil 1 teaspoon of one herb or all three in 2 cups of water. I drink this twice daily.

How to determine the calories you need.

Before you attempt fat reduction, you need to know how to calculate your daily intake of calories. This is important. To lose fat safely and preserve as much muscle possible, aim to burn at least 1 pound (0.45 kilograms) of fat, which is 3,500 calories per week to make a significant impact. Depending on your size, if you cut 500 to 1000 calories a day from your diet, you could lose 1 to 2 pounds per week. For example, you are female, 5'6" and weigh 160lbs. To maintain your current weight, your estimated caloric needs may be 1,750 per day. To determine your caloric needs, use the calorie calculator to estimate the number of daily calories your body needs to maintain your current weight. Refer to this link:

https://www.mayoclinic.org/healthy-lifestyle/weight-loss/in-depth/calorie-calculator/itt-20402304.

Now, if you want to lose 1 pound a week, decrease your daily caloric needs of 1,750 by 500, which would amount to a daily caloric consumption of 1,250. Then you would want to design your meal plan to incorporate those calories. Keep in mind that you may find out that this intake is not suitable for your level of activity and it may not cause any reduction. If you are not sure, this is an excellent time to consult with a health professional or personal trainer.

Although it is necessary to have a calorie deficit for body fat loss, there is no need to starve yourself, hoping that you will lose weight quickly. Unfortunately, that is exactly what you will lose, weight, and not just fat. Not only will you be miserable, but you run the risk of Grandma pestering you—"you are what you eat—nibbling on that lettuce leaf." She may be right. You can end up with a soft marshmallow muscle frame. Not only that, but this can also encourage binge eating when you are hungry. Depriving yourself of food can also slow down your metabolism, and may cause inadequate processing of nutrients.

Once you have determined your daily caloric requirements, you can design a balanced-meal plan to help you achieve fat loss. ***What is a well-balanced meal?*** A balanced meal comprises the essential nutrients from different food groups (in adequate quantity) for the body to function optimally. It includes carbohydrates, healthy fats, vitamins and minerals, protein, and fibre. The required amounts of nutrients depend on an individual need.

It is important to remember that both complex starches and simple sugars are worth limiting—especially simple sugars, but do not get carried away because they both have a place in nutrition and the digestion cycle.

The difference between the two will help in designing your fat-loss strategy.

Starches are present in a variety of foods, including foods with high nutrition content. However, all starches are not created equal:

Nutrition-rich carbs: some of which are Quinoa, peas, beans, oats, and root vegetables such as turnips, eddoes, yams, and sweet potatoes. These starches contain dietary fibre and are great for a fat-loss meal plan. Such carbs digest gradually, which will keep you feeling fuller longer because it slows the conversion of carbs to glucose (sugar).

Refined carbs: these are white flour sources such as pasta, white bread, and pastries. Such starches are not suitable for a fat-loss meal plan. These carbs go directly to the bloodstream and quickly turn to sugar, which causes the blood sugar level to rise. It may cause insulin resistance and could lead to weight gain.

Nutrition-rich sugars: they are raw fresh fruits low in calories; some of which are grapefruits, berries, kiwi, cherries, apples, melons, and avocados. Though these fruits contain sugar, they do not raise blood sugar levels drastically, and are more likely to support fat loss.

Refined fruit sugars: they lack little or no nutritional value. Usually, they are found in carbonated (soft) beverages, table sugar, juice concentrates, fruit juices, sports drinks and other refined or processed products. Like refined starches, they allow for sugar to pass into the bloodstream rapidly. The direct passage causes an increase in blood sugar that provides high energy. When the blood sugar level decreases, there is a sudden drop in energy—a sugar crash. These types of sugars are not ideal for fat loss.

How your meal plan could help body fat loss:

When drafting your meal plan, take into consideration your pre-workout and post-workout meals. They are both important for losing fat.

A pre-workout meal will help to provide energy for your up-coming session. It is best to consume the meal one or two hours before exercising. About 20 to 30 minutes before your training, you may have a protein or carb drink such as a smoothie, snack on a banana and hydrate with water. It can make a huge difference for maximum workout intensity—lifting more pounds and engaging additional reps. Here are some ideas for such a meal: turkey, chicken, tuna, egg whites, sweet potatoes.

A post-workout meal is also essential because after a workout, your stored energy is depleted. This meal refuels the body for recovery. It helps replenish and repair muscles and prevents protein breakdown. After your workout have easy-to-digest liquid nutrients, such as a protein/carb recovery drink: chocolate milk, protein, or avocado smoothies are good sources of fuel until you can consume a balanced meal, which will feed your body with nutrients. Here are some meal ideas: chicken breast, beef, fish, fruits, vegetables, whole-grains, legumes, sweet potatoes and diary.

Drafting a healthy meal plan is easy, but **note that eating healthy does not cause you to lose fat; you have to create a calorie deficit for fat loss.** There is no hard and fast rule. We all have different appetite levels, lifestyles, schedules, preferences, activity levels, or may have individual health requirements. Design a meal plan that works for your fitness goals.

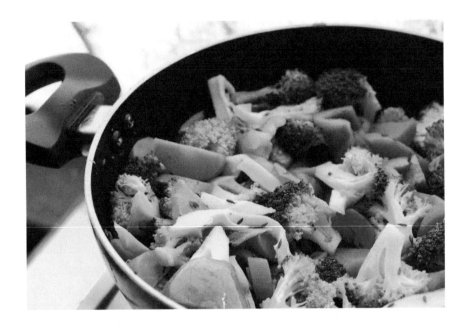

Non-Vegetarian

Monday

Breakfast:

1 boiled egg
1 slice 100% whole grain
bread toasted
1 cup black coffee

Snack
Home-made veggie pack
5 Almonds nuts

Lunch
Veggie salad
3 oz. turkey breast
1 cup strawberries

Snack

Home-made veggie pack
1 cup sliced strawberries/blueberies

Dinner

1 Salmon steak
1 cup steamed broccoli
1 cup mashed sweet potatoes

Vegetarian / Vegan

Monday

Breakfast:

1 cup oats
4 tbsp yogurt
¼ chopped apple with blueberries

Snack
Home-made veggie pack
5 Almond nuts

Lunch
Veggie Burrito salad bowl
1 bottle water

Snack

Home-made veggie pack
1 cup sliced strawberries/ blueberries

Dinner

1 cup quinoa with beans
1 cup tofu
2 cups steamed vegetables
1 cup mashed sweet potatoes

**Design a similar meal plan for each day of the
week, regardless of you eating preferences.**

Here is a link for healthy meal-plan ideas:

https://www.kraftwhatscooking.ca/recipes/recipes-1000001.

If you pre-cook a variety of meals, it will prevent you from ordering in when you are tired from a hard day's work. All you would have to do is warm up the already-cooked meal.

Your meal plan should guide you on what type of foods to purchase. Before grocery shopping, go through a nutritional inventory of your kitchen cupboards, pantry, and refrigerator, and remove all unhealthy fat-gaining foods. If these products are not around, you will not be tempted to eat them. You can reference to the Appendix for staple food items for your pantry and refrigerator.

At the grocery store, you are there to purchase healthy-fat foods, fruits, vegetables and grains. This is unquestionably one of the best ways to make healthier dietary alterations. Note that although organic harvest may be more beneficial, it does not have to be your objective for eating healthy, especially if your budget does not allow for such purchases. You could still get many benefits from non-organic produce. Also, know that going to the grocery store on an empty stomach can be a fat trap. You roaming the aisles to figure out where that scent of cheese is coming from. Always make sure you have eaten. If not, you may end up demo snacking products, encouraging you to purchase unwanted items.

Note that because you have purchased healthy foods, you might think it is all right to overeat. Remember, your stomach can only hold so much food—regardless of quality. If the rest of the food cannot be metabolized and absorbed, it can turn into fat. So avoid checking in the cupboards and refrigerator time and again, trying to find something to eat; there is nothing in there that you have not seen the last time you opened that door. Also, refrain from constantly checking the scale too. Look in the mirror more than at the scale.

Food to consider for fat loss:

When trying to lose fat, do not cut corners when consuming meals, for example, consuming pre-packaged processed foods that save meal-time preparation. Preparing your own meals can be healthier; you could save money and your meals would not be handled with unhealthy preservatives and additives.

Consuming whole grains and whole foods is a fundamental part of any fat-loss program. **Whole grains** comprise the whole grain kernel, unrefined. They are rich in nutrients, some of which are magnesium, selenium, vitamins, iron and other plant benefits; they contain antioxidants that are not present in vegetables or fruits; they are high in fibre and low in fat, which contributes to fat loss; they speed up the metabolism, which helps to burn calories. Some whole grains include brown rice, wild rice, oats, quinoa, millet, and buckwheat. Whole grain comes in starches too, such as bread, which many people love to eat. The starch makes it taste good. Although there is nothing wrong with consuming bread, refrain from buying bread that has been refined or enhanced. They may have little to no nutritional value. Some breads you might want to purchase are sprouted whole grain, flaxseed, sourdough, or gluten free. Know your bread. One of many healthier options is **100% whole grain bread** because the entire grain is intact with all its nutrients.

Whole foods come in a natural state or as close to it as possible. They include raw, fresh fruits and vegetables, legumes, and whole-grain. Healthy whole food snacking is a great way to help you burn calories. A good practice outside your meal plan is to always carry a snack pack of celery, carrots, nuts, chopped fruits, unsalted pumpkin seeds, strips of bell peppers, or some low-calorie nutritional bits readily available for when you feel peckish. The unhealthy food cravings will soon end with this little change in the habit of carrying your own tidbits around.

Although chewing sugarless gum is not a typical snack, it can help stifle your ravenous inclination to eat. A gum that I have tried is called Xylitol because it also helps to kill bacteria in the mouth. It is mainly found in health food stores. Gum ends up giving your mouth something to do, saving you from a nibbling crisis.

In addition, protein is vital to the body regardless of whether you are vegetarian or vegan. While plant-based foods have a high nutritional value and are necessary for good health, so is animal protein. It is a great source of essential amino acids not obtainable from just plants. Lean meats and fish varities are crucial for fat loss because it has a satiating effect.

Foods to avoid for fat loss

The foods you consume, however delicious, will have a significant effect on fat loss. Refraining from calorie-dense foods is best. As already mentioned, calories are not the only factors to be considered. If you only consume low-calorie foods, (with the exception of greens) they may lack adequate nutrients, which could leave you hungry. This can cause you to indulge in constant snacking to satisfy hunger pangs.

There are certain foods to eliminate from your diet when trying to lose body fat. It is almost impossible to list *all* the foods to avoid, but there are three major foods to cut from your diet after detoxification:

1. **Refined sugars:** white sugar, high fructose corn syrup.

2. **Refined carbs:** wheat products.

3. **Unhealthy Fats:** vegetable oils.

Removing these three foods would help stimulate significant fat loss. Remember, it is also important to exercise.

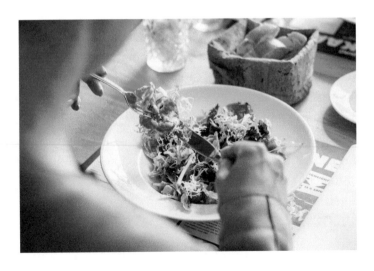

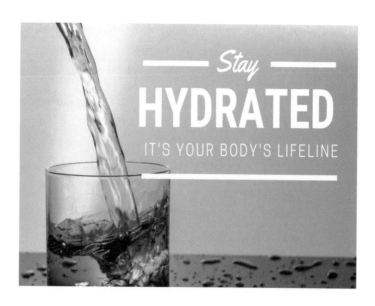

Drinks to burn calories:

There are many liquids you can consume to help burn calories. To name a few of them, there are:

1. Green Tea.
2. Ginger Tea
3. Black Coffee
4. Black Tea
5. Apple Cider Vinegar
   *add 1 tablespoon of apple cider vinegar to 1 cup of warm water.
6. Water
7. Coconut Water
8. High-Protein Drinks
9. Broth
10. Almond Milk
11. Skim Milk

Avoid commercial fruit juices—do not be fooled by the label showing appealing whole fruits as "natural fruit juice." They are just as "natural" like the "natural" pictures some celebrities post on Instagram. Do not always believe what you see. Such juices may not contain the quality product as advertised. Commercial fruit juices are usually made from concentrate and are loaded with added sugar. Further, these fruit juices are not a good substitution for eating fresh whole fruits.

In addition, leafy green smoothies are nourishing, delicious, and easy to make. Leafy vegetables do not have fat; they are water soluble. They do not contribute to body fat. One could start with a spinach smoothie.

Also, drinking coffee could help you lose body fat. It is not the coffee that contributes to gaining the pounds; it is the creamers and sugars. If you like coffee, try to acquire a taste for drinking it black; it would not adversely impact fat loss.

Burn calories while stressed:

"Stress is not the advocate towards your goal.
Positive thinking gives credence to your aspirations."
Avaneil John

Stress can help you gain weight or lose weight, which varies for different people. Sometimes when we are heavily stressed, weight loss can occur, but this is unintentional. It is the intentional fat loss that will provide a sound reduction of fat. However, the reverse could happen. Stress or anger may lead you to engage in comfort eating. Comfort foods will not decrease the stress but can work against you because you are likely to put on extra pounds. In such circumstances, find an activity that will curb the desire for comfort eating. You can go for a walk; you would burn some calories instead of eating them.

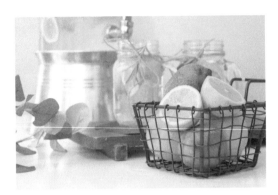

Cheat day for weight loss:

Once you have been on the journey of stabilizing your weight, you deserve a cheat meal day. Having a regularly scheduled cheat day each week can be good for weight loss by preventing binges, reducing cravings, providing a mental break from dieting, and boosting metabolism—if it is done in a healthy way.

Although some cheat-meals may be refined, I do not believe in eating healthy all the time. I do not deprive myself of a cheat day for pizza, ice-cream, or a burger once a week. You can eat what you like on a cheat day but consume smaller portions. Moderation is key to effective fat loss. Stay in control and do not periodically binge! After your cheat meal, you must have the willpower to get right back on your regular healthy eating habits immediately. This is a test of your self-discipline and determination. If you do not trust your willpower, do not have a cheat meal.

If you are dining at a restaurant on your cheat day, refrain from nibbling on the complimentary starters—you know—the white-flour garlic-bread basket or dried/fried chips. They are empty fat-gaining calories. They want to destroy the illusion of being slim.

Now that you have some idea of how to control your caloric intake, I will show you how a workout program is a great and necessary complement.

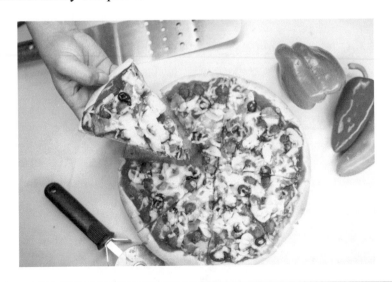

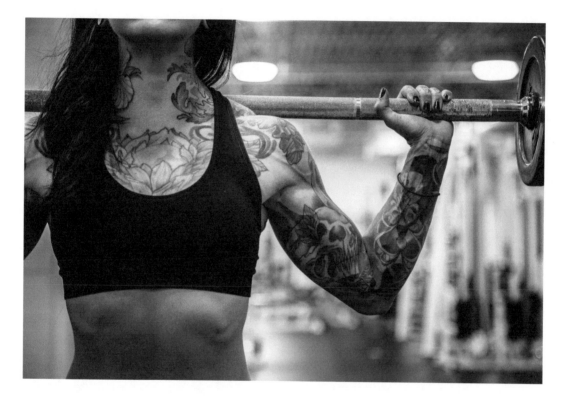

In this section, you will know the components of a workout, how to design a program, required equipment, and support system. Designing a workout program comprises four components:

Warm up

Many individuals think a warm up is not an essential part of the exercise. They are wrong. The main purpose of a warm up is to prevent injuries such as muscle pull or joint injury. A warm up mentally prepares your body for the upcoming exercises. Some benefits of warm-up exercises include increasing the body's temperature, heart rate, and blood circulation,

Some examples of warm-up exercises are on-the-spot jogging, skipping, jumping jacks, or swinging of the body's extremities.

Strength training for weight loss

Strength training can lead to fat loss; the more muscle you have, the more calories you could burn. This training is one of the critical ways to burn fat and build muscles. Engaging multiple (compound/full-body exercise) muscle groups helps to speed up metabolism. Strength training exercises can be done at home, outdoors, or at the gym. Your choices are many, and some of your options could include using little or no weights: bodyweight, resistance bands, free weights, and weight machines.

Cardio

One of the many questions I have been asked is, *"What kind of cardio exercises can one do to lose weight?"* There is no specific cardio method that is classified as the best. There are many forms of cardio activities like aerobics, treadmill, biking, running, elliptical, or free-style cardio.

However, one of the cardio exercises that can maximize burning fat is High-Intensity Interval Training (HIIT). The concept of HIIT refers to alternating frequently between low intensity to high-intensity workout periods. For example, you may sprint for 30 seconds and walk for 60 seconds, then repeat the cycle. HIIT is a great exercise to include in your plan. It can also apply to your weight-training program. See HIIT workout examples on page 19.

Stretching

Stretching is an actual form of exercise and should be a part of your exercise plan. If you do not stretch your muscles, your range of motion over time may become limited. Stretching relaxes the muscles worked, increases blood circulation, improves the range of motion and flexibility. One of the best times to stretch is right after your cardio exercise when your muscles are warm and pliable. It is also a perfect exercise strategy for cooling down.

How to design a simple program

Before designing your physical fitness programs, know what is needed. Would you need a workout buddy? Will you be using thera-bands, strength bands, weights or just bodyweight?

Design exercises suitable for your lifestyle and fitness level. There is no point to a workout program if you are frequently missing your workout. As a beginner, it is not wise to design an advanced workout. The exercises may not be suited to your needs, but you can always design one for your level and specificity. Note that your program must include all components. The design can be as simple as the examples below:

Full Body Workout				
Days	**Strength Training**	**Exercises**	**Sets**	**Reps**
			3	8-10
Monday	Total body weight	Pull-ups, push-ups, Squats to overhead press		
Tuesday	Interval cardio Weight training	Jogging, skipping Core, chest, triceps, biking.		
Wednesday	Rest Day	This can even be a Yoga mindful session		
Design your workout for each day of the week, regardless of the days you choose to workout.				

Alternating Body Workout							
Exercises	**Set 3 - 4**	**Reps 8 - 12**	**Weeks**				**Rest Days 2 - 3**
			W 1	W 2	W 3	W 4	Comments
Dumbbell Bench Press Dumbbell Flys Hanging Knee Raises Stability Ball Plank			✓				
Squats Reverse Lunges Hamstring Curls Leg Extensions Calf Raises Shoulders				✓			
Design your workout for each week. Include at least 2 body parts each workout.							

Examples: Simple High-Intensity Interval Training (HIIT) workout plan to help lose body fat:

- **Warm Up**: 10 minutes.

- **Intervals**: 2 minutes at 85-90% of near max heart rate (working out very hard).

- 3 minutes at 60% of max heart rate (light workload).

- 2 minutes at 85-90% of near max heart rate. (Working out very hard)

- 3 minutes at 60% of max heart rate. (light workload).

- **Cool Down:** 10 minutes.

Total Workout Time: 30 minutes.

Another HIIT workout could be as simple as this method below:

High-Intensity Interval Training

- 30-second sprint / 60 seconds light jog

- 30-second speed walk / 60 seconds slow walk

- 30 seconds of activity / 30-second rest (next level)

These variations can be repeated at least 3 to 4 times, then increasing the distance or intensity each week can burn a considerable amount of fat.

Also, there are great alternative venues for working out. Not everyone prefers conventional training by going to the gym. You may prefer the convenience of your home or outdoors. If this is the case, you can visit https://www.xquisitefitness.com/ for such exercises. Some other unconventional options for working out can be gardening, mowing the lawn, engaging in home renovations, and climbing the stairwell (as opposed to taking the elevator). These exercises keep you moving and help in the toning of the muscles.

Know that there comes a point in your workout when you may reach a plateau. Your body does not require the same amount of energy—your progress has stalled. This occurs when the calories you burn (energy) equals the calories you consume or a repeated workout regime. Do not be discouraged—keep up the motivation. You may experience several plateaus in your journey; it is normal. A plateau can be a good thing if you are satisfied with your weight. If you are not, here are some tips that may help to stimulate fat loss in progress: you can rev up the physical intensity of your workout by attempting new exercises; adding more days to workout; changing food options or decreasing your nutritional intake—provided that you do not go below 1,200 calories. Calories below this amount can cause constant hunger or external and internal dysfunction.

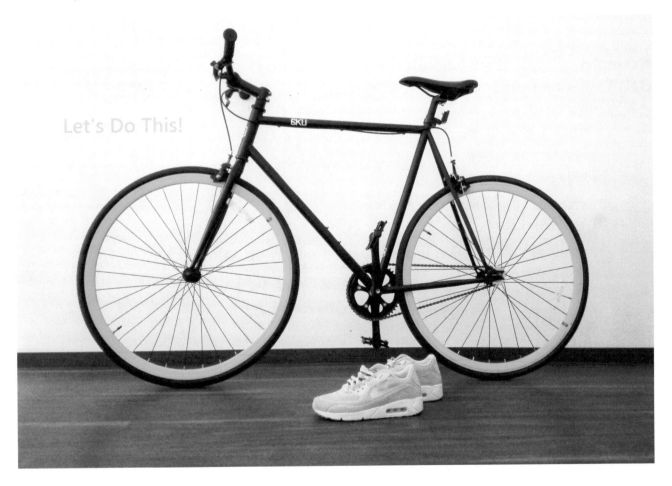

AVANEIL JOHN

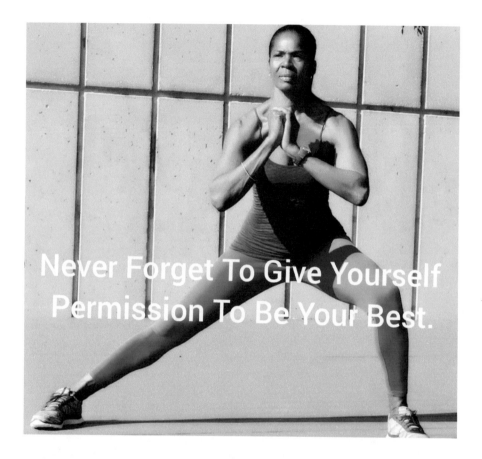

Never Forget To Give Yourself Permission To Be Your Best.

Sometimes working out alone can be daunting and can cause a lack of motivation. If this is the case, a workout buddy is essential. A workout buddy allows you to be part of a team. But ensure what each buddy wants to achieve from the workout. Not all fitness partners are created equal. Your partner may be at a more advanced fitness level. The difference in capabilities can hold each other back.

Having someone with similar objectives engage in exercises with you can lead to a bolstering of each other's motivation and realization that you are both destined for success. If you do not have a workout partner, you may find someone by asking your friends, family, or you could join online fat-loss chat groups.

Benefits of having a workout buddy:

- **Motivation**: Despite your best intention, you may sometimes lack motivation. A workout buddy can push you through the exercise. This will help you achieve your goals.

- **Accountability:** Sometimes you may not want to work out. But if someone is relying on you, the commitment is greater; you are more likely to make the effort.

- **Coaching:** a personal trainer can be a good work-out buddy. The trainer can motivate you and ensure that you are doing the exercises correctly.

- **Friendly competition:** You can set challenging, achievable goals, such as who will walk 3 miles on the treadmill. The defeated individual takes the winner to a movie.

- **Emotional Bond:** exercising with a partner can be great for relationships. The support and sociability can help in bonding more closely with each other.

- **Having fun:** Working out is supposed to be fun. The more you have fun, the more likely you are to commit to your workout plan.

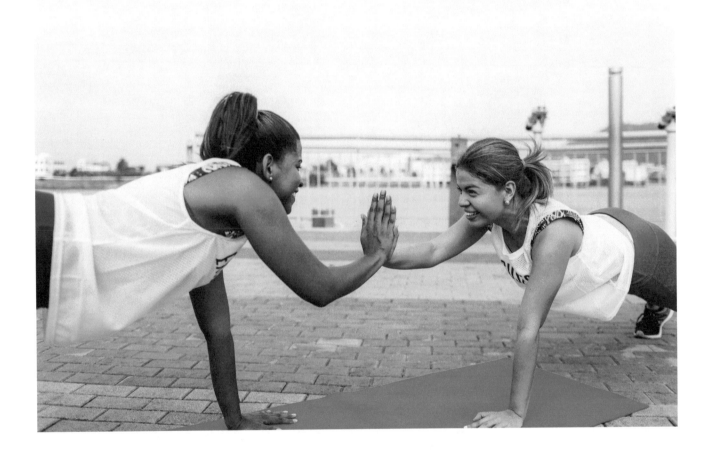

WEIGHT MAINTENANCE - KEEPING IT OFF!

Calories needed to maintain the current weight:

Fat loss and weight maintenance are two different processes. At this stage, you need not focus solely on dieting, but on exercises to help in maintaining the new weight. Losing fat, as challenging as it may be, makes you look and feel fantastic. Your success is unquestionable because it makes you feel great. Your efforts have paid off, but the journey is not over.

Attaining your new weight may have been difficult for you, and maintaining it may be just as, or more challenging. At this phase, many people fail because once the targeted weight is reached, they think it is mission accomplished. This is a delicate stage because your body would keep trying to regain weight. If you help it by going back to older eating habits, your efforts would have been wasted. This is the reason to make a slow transition to weight maintenance.

Maintain the same mindset you acquired to lose body fat and apply it to this stage. Also, you must know how many calories are needed to maintain your current weight and what exercise methods can be used for sustaining it. Note that it is not uncommon for some people to keep losing extra pounds surpassing their goal. If this should happen, add to your meal plan about 100 to 150 calories of healthy low-calorie foods. Do this for one or two weeks and monitor the intake closely until you reach your desired weight again.

To determine the required calories to sustain the target weight, use the online calorie calculator link provided earlier. Now, design a well-balanced meal plan to allow for the needed calories. Your meal plan should be high in protein, low in carbs, and have good fats, vitamins and minerals. **Do not** focus on dieting.

Stay active to maintain current weight:

Exercise is vital for the maintenance of weight. You have to balance the same amount of exercise output to caloric intake. This is the stage when you can pay regular attention to the scale. It allows you to detect any weight gain in time to keep you on track.

To maintain weight, physical-activity calories may need to be 1,400 to 2,000 depending on the demands of your workout. Engage in 60 to 90 minutes of moderate to vigorous exercises three to four times weekly. Eating a healthy well-balanced meal and exercising would help you control the current weight.

It takes physical and mental exertion to push ahead and defeat obstacles. Taking action by venturing with no hesitation may be difficult initially, but attaining your goal will eventually be your reward.

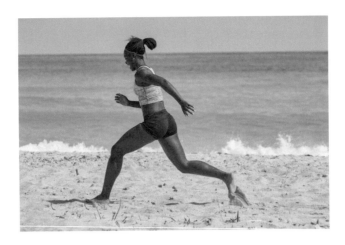

Seven main tips to consider when maintaining weight:

1. Weigh yourself regularly: this will help you notice any additional pounds.

2. Set warning weight: on the scale, you noticed you have gained two pounds. Act immediately to lose it by going back to your fat-loss plan.

3. Determine weight-gain triggers: Going to an elaborate dinner? Eat your own-designed meal before you attend the function. This way, you will be full and less likely to binge, but watch what you nibble on.

4. Physical activity: exercise regularly to maintain your current weight. The more intense your workout, the more calories you will burn.

5. Accountability: keep yourself accountable to your new weight—keep your eyes on the prize.

6. Consistency: to maintain your new weight, be consistent with your daily exercises. You will reap the benefits.

7. Nutrition: Again, lessen or avoid refined and processed starches and table sugars.

Summary

Achieving fat loss should not be an arbitrary process. To engage in effective fat loss, you have to understand what is required mentally and physically. You will easily sustain your goals if you plan for the process of fat loss.

There are no magic tricks or pills that will cause immediate results. Body fat reduction is a gradual process. Patience is the key. Quick diet plans may cause more harm to your goal than good.

Nutrition is a key aspect of fat loss. Eating healthy foods prevent consuming extra calories from processed foods, which will help you achieve your goal. To get in shape, do not focus on cardiovascular (cardio) exercises alone. Incorporate strength training as part of your program. Building muscle will help in burning calories. The reason being is that muscle burns calories from fat.

It is important to understand that both exercise and nutrition are the key components to any successful fat-loss improvement. Once you make lifestyle changes as a feature of your get-healthy plan, you will discover more ways on your own to approach getting fit.

To maintain your new physique, keep empowering and challenging yourself through weight training. You will look and feel great!

Fat-Loss Pantry/Cupboard and Fridge Staples

Beans and Legumes	Red beans, black beans, black-eyed peas, chickpeas, lentils.
Beverages	Plain water, almond milk, coconut water, coconut milk, lemon/lime water.
Fruits	Avocado, banana, mango, strawberries, blueberries, pineapple, grapefruit, lemon, lime, kiwi, apples.
Grains	Brown Rice, quinoa, oats, amanathan, millet, chia seeds, buckwheat.
Lean Meat Products	Chicken, beef, turkey, vegan or vegetarian meats, tuna stake, wild salmon, (canned sardines, canned tuna – emergency options).
Nuts and Seeds	Brazil nuts, almonds, walnuts, cashews, pumpkin seeds, hemp seeds, flaxseeds.
Oils	Avocado oil, coconut oil, extra virgin olive oil.
Other food Staples	Honey, nut butters, Tahini, hummus, honey Dijon mustard, eggs, yogurt, pickles, grape tomatoes.
Powders	Protein, moringa, maca, cacao.
Vegetables	Broccoli, cauliflower, asparagus, spinach, kale, mixed spring greens, cucumber, celery, sweet potatoes, bell peppers, mushrooms, onion, garlic.

ABOUT THE AUTHOR

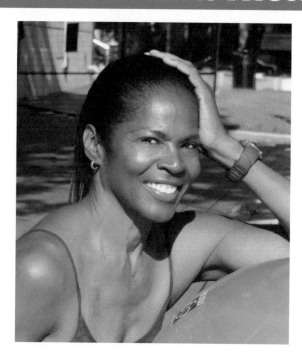

Avaneil John is a certified strength-and-conditioning personal trainer with over 11 years of experience. She is a Hons. Physiotherapist Assistant. Avaneil has studied holistic nutrition, being a weight-loss specialist in the field, and is also a weight-management consultant.

Avaneil is the owner and operator of Xquisite Fitness in Toronto. She has successfully used many of the principles provided to facilitate fat loss in her clients.

The book came about because she wants to guide and inspire readers who are not under the guidance of a coach to help themselves for attaining and maintaining fat loss. The fat-loss process would help them to practice a lifestyle that is healthier from her experiences and insights as a personal trainer.

"You cannot buy good health to live a healthier lifestyle.
But you can create a healthier lifestyle to live in good health. "
Avaneil John

Printed in the United States
by Baker & Taylor Publisher Services